Effective Techniques To Eliminate Bad Breath Immediately

By Dannie Elwins

Copyright © 2009 By Dannie Elwins

No part of this publication may be reproduced or transmitted in any form or by any means, mechanical or electronic, including photocopying and recording, or by any information storage and retrieval system, without permission in writing from author or publisher.

OBLIGATORY LEGAL NOTICE: While all attempts have been made to verify information provided in this publication, neither the Author nor the Publisher assumes any responsibility for errors, omissions, or contrary interpretation of the subject matter herein. Any perceived slights of specific persons, peoples, or organizations is unintentional.

This publication is an information product, and is not intended for use as a source of legal, medical, accounting, or tax advice. Information contained herein may be subject to varying national, state, and/or local laws or regulations. All users are advised to retain the services of competent professionals for legal, medical, accounting, or tax advice.

The purchaser or reader of this publication assumes responsibility for the use of these materials and information, including adherence to all applicable laws and regulations, federal, state, and local, governing professional licensing, business practices, advertising, and all other aspects of doing business in the United States or any other jurisdiction in the world.

No guarantees are made. Publisher reserves the right to make changes. If you can't accept these terms, kindly return product. The Author and Publisher assume no responsibility or liability whatsoever on the behalf of any purchaser or reader of these materials.

Printed in the United States of America.

ISBN: 978-0-557-15437-1

Table of Contents

What Is Bad Breath? 5
    How To Check For Bad Breath 5
Causes Of Bad Breath 6
Getting Rid Of Bad Breath 10
    Oral Hygiene 10
    Foods 13
    Vitamins and Supplements 14
    Digestive System 14
    Herbal Remedies 15
    Chinese Herbs 17
    Breath Spray 18
    Over The Counter Medications (OTC) 18
    Using Flaxseed For Bad Breath 19
    Quick Remedies For Bad Breath 20
When You Should Seek Medical Assistance 22
How Smokers Can Get Rid Of Bad Breath 24
How To Prevent Or Stop Bad Breath 26
    Flossing 26
    Brushing 28
    Using Tongue Brushing To Get Rid Of Bad Breath 28
How To Help Others That Have Bad Breath 30
    Children That Have Bad Breath 30
    The Date With Bad Breath 31

How To Tell A Friend Or Family Member 33

Resources... 34

What Is Bad Breath?

Bad breath is when there is an unpleasant odor that usually comes from the mouth. When people exhale, the odor comes out. Not only is it a health issue, but it is also a social issue as well. People get turned off by those that have bad breath when they open their mouth.

How To Check For Bad Breath

There are different ways to determine whether or not you have bad breath. Here are some ways that you can do this:

- This is about the easiest way for you to find out if you have bad breath. Breathe on the back of your hands. You will automatically smell the odor as it comes out of your mouth. This can determine how your breath really smells.

- Did you know that saliva has an odor? Well, if you didn't, you do now. You hope that when you conduct this test that your breath will not have a foul odor. To do this, you will slightly lick your wrist or the back of your hand.

  Give it a few seconds and then take a whiff. If you don't smell anything, then you should be ok. If you do, check with your dentist and get help.

- You can use a spoon or a tongue scraper to test your breath. Scrape your tongue at the front and back. Do each area one at a time. Smell the area in question on the spoon or the scraper and see how it smells. If it is a foul smell, then you may have chronic bad breath (halitosis).

- Check to see if you have any black spots on your teeth. If you do, it could be a sign that you may have bad breath. You may end up having tooth and gum problems that could also lead to bad breath due to bacteria that has formed.

Consult with your dentist to provide treatment to those areas that are affected so you can head off a potential bout of bad breath.

Halitosis is when you have chronic bad breath. Now that's worse when it's chronic. Whether it happens a few times or it's a continuous problem, people should find ways to get rid of it. As for the cause of bad breath, there are different reasons why it's happening.

Causes Of Bad Breath

- **Food** – When you eat, the food particles that remain in and around your teeth can cause an odor in your mouth. Of course, everyone knows that eating onions (raw ones, especially) and garlic are some of the worst culprits.

  After you have digested these foods and smelly oils, they penetrate through your blood. Then they travel to your lungs and come up in your breath when you open your mouth. It's possible to have an onion or garlic smell for at least three days.

- **Dental issues** – Periodontal disease, which occurs from poor dental hygiene, can also cause bad breath. Food particles will remain in your mouth if you don't brush and floss daily. You'll probably have to brush and floss several times a day. If the food particles remain in your mouth, they will absorb bacteria.

  You may experience plaque on your teeth. If you don't brush your teeth properly or not enough, the plaque can mess with your gums. You can end up getting gingivitis and tooth decay. Pockets can form between your teeth and gums. This condition is called periodonitis. Peridonitis can cause the bad breath to linger.

- **Dry mouth** – The inside of your mouth should always be moist with saliva. Saliva is used to clean your mouth. If you don't have any saliva circulating on the inside, dead cells will gather on your tongue. They can also come on your cheeks and gums. This condition is called dry mouth.

Once the dead cells accumulate, they start to deteriorate, causing a foul odor inside of the mouth. This condition usually happens when a person is sleeping. If you sleep with your mouth open, you are more prone to get dry mouth. When you wake up in the morning, dry mouth can also cause what is known as "morning breath."

- **Chronic diseases** – Certain chronic lung ailments such as infections and abscesses can emit foul odors as you open your mouth. If you have chronic kidney failure, you could have an odor that smells like urine.

A fishy odor could be the result of chronic liver ailments. Those that have diabetes have a fruity odor. Also, some stomach ailments have been linked to bad breath.

- **Nose and throat infections** – A person can also have bad breath from allergies. Sinus infections cause a nasal discharge. It goes from the back of the throat and trickles downward. This can cause a foul odor. You can also have bad breath if you have upper respiratory ailments in which you cough up mucus.

- **Tobacco** – If you smoke cigarettes, it causes your mouth to be dry. Smoking causes an unpleasant odor after you have puffed on a cigarette. If you are a smoker, there is a greater chance for you to get periodontal disease, which would be a double whammy because that also causes bad breath.

- **Extreme dieting** – If you use a special diet or fasting to lose weight, you may have a fruity breath. This is a result of developing ketoacidosis, which is when the chemicals break down while you're fasting.

- **Milk** – If you find out that you're intolerant of milk, then you'll have to get rid of it. You can develop bad breath if you're consuming milk or dairy products that you can't digest.

- **Alcohol** – Drinking alcohol can cause health issues with your digestive system. It also causes dry mouth, which can lead to bad breath.

- **Stress** – You probably would have never thought that stress could cause bad breath, but it can. When you're stressed out, your digestive system is affected, which triggers bad breath.

Even with normal fresh breath, it could eventually transform into halitosis. Here are some other things that can cause bad breath:

- Cavities
- Dentures
- Drugs
- Insulin
- Gingivitis
- Vitamin Supplements
- Tonsils that catch food particles
- Cancer of the throat or mouth
- HIV infection
- Dehydration

There are solutions that you can try that can improve the quality of your breath. You can also use these to prevent bad breath.

Getting Rid Of Bad Breath

Oral Hygiene

Regular oral hygiene is very important for your dental health as well as your regular health. With oral hygiene, you need to focus on three key areas of your mouth: the teeth, gums and tongue. It's important to brush and floss your teeth at least twice a day.

- Make sure that you brush your teeth after you eat. If you work away from home, take a toothbrush with you so you can brush after you eat lunch.

- You need to use floss at least once a day, maybe more. Flossing helps to remove food particles that are stuck in your teeth. It also helps to remove plaque. It is very important to get rid of any plaque that is on your teeth because not only can it cause periodontal disease, it can also cause heart disease and other heart ailments.

- As weird as it may sound, brushing your teeth can remove dead cells from your tongue. It also works to remove any leftover food particles and bacteria. To do this, use a toothbrush with a soft bristle or a tongue scraper.

  Go as far back into the mouth as you can. Try it without gagging. You will find that most of the bacteria are settled toward the back.

- If you wear dentures, make sure you clean them thoroughly. They should be cleaned at least once a day.

- When you brush your teeth, use a brush with small bristles. Change out your toothbrush at least every four months.

- See your dentist on a regular basis. You should have your teeth or dentures cleaned and checked twice a year, if not more.

- If you have cavities, make an appointment with your dentist to have them filled. Cavities are also an opening to allow bacteria in, which in turn can cause bad breath.

- After you've eaten breakfast, use a water pik to clean your mouth as well as get rid of any food particles left behind.

- Swish water in your mouth after you eat a meal. You will be able to get rid of some of the food particles that were stuck in your teeth. Using a solution mixed with water, you can also treat periodontal disease.

- You can also choose to use natural oral hygiene remedies to get rid of bad breath. Using baking soda and hydrogen peroxide can do wonders. If you really want to sanitize your mouth, use a natural remedy by adding some antiseptic tree oil or eucalyptus oil.

  You only want to add a little oil on your toothbrush. You can also go to the health food store to get natural toothpaste remedies.

- To sanitize your toothbrush, place it in a container of hydrogen peroxide to keep your toothbrush bacteria-free. When you get ready to brush your teeth, rinse the toothbrush very well.

- Work to keep your mouth free of food particles, especially those that get stuck in your teeth and pocket areas. Try not to make it a habit to eat spicy foods that have onions and garlic in them.

- Put a small portion of fresh parsley or a small mint (sugarless) in your mouth. You may notice an improvement in your breath.

- Drink lots of water to keep the inside of your mouth moist. You can also produce saliva by chewing sugarless gum or candy. If your mouth is always dry, you can get a prescription of artificial saliva preparation or an oral prescription that produces saliva in your mouth.

- People use tongue scrapers to get rid of bad breath. They can be purchased at pharmacies and they come in different shapes and sizes. The scraper is placed at the back of the tongue. The tongue and the scraper are bought forward. This can be repeated as many times as needed.

Some people say that this method helps a little to eliminate bad breath. There are others who prefer using a toothbrush to remove the bacteria from the tongue. It's ok to use a tongue scraper, but it's even better to implement dental hygiene on a regular basis. Make sure along with brushing your teeth that you also brush your tongue after you eat.

- Keeping saliva in your mouth keeps bacteria away by drinking lots of water. Try not to get the mouthwash at the drugstore. That mouthwash is usually concentrated with alcohol. Alcohol dries your mouth and can produce bacteria.

Also, mouthwash that contains more than 25% of alcohol is believed to contribute to oral cancer. Look for a mouthwash that has a mixture of at least half hydrogen peroxide and half water. Take a little bit and swish it in your mouth for about 30 seconds.
Since bacteria are what cause the bad breath to form, you have to counteract it with things that don't promote it. Many people don't know this, but the bacteria lives underneath your tongue.

You can also find bacteria on your tonsils and your throat. This means that you cannot easily get rid of it. So, in order to combat that, people use mouthwash that contains alcohol. In turn, you end up getting dry mouth and more bacteria to form.

- If you are a smoker, learn to kick the habit. Tobacco related products are not good for you health wise, even with the bad breath.

- Avoid consuming liquids that have a bad smell. The smell can linger in your mouth. Stick with water and go easy on juice and liquor.

- If you don't gargle, now is a good time to start. There may be some difficult places
where bacteria can creep in while you're sleeping. Do it for at least 30 seconds each   morning and get as close to the bottom of your throat as you

can. Make sure to rinse after you've finished getting all of the bacteria and other elements out.

- Since salt is used to kill bacteria, mixing it with water can help to eliminate bad breath and halitosis.

Foods

There are certain types of foods that you consume that can be a culprit to bad breath. Food that is high in fat, meats, foods loaded with sugar, specialty spices and dairy products. Foods that contain acid produce bacteria in your mouth.

When you eat foods with a lot of fat and protein, they may not digest in your system properly. People that have difficulty digesting meat and dairy products can end up with bad breath.

Here are some suggestions regarding foods when it comes to bad breath:

- Make sure to include fruits and vegetables that are rich with antioxidants. This would include leafy greens, berries, broccoli and cabbage. These foods help to keep you healthy and to keep bad breath from occurring.

- You can also eat yogurt that is sugar-free and has a live culture. This helps to keep away bacteria that are responsible for causing halitosis.

- Foods that are loaded with sugar pose a problem because the sugar affects the back of the throat.

- In addition to onions and garlic, spices such as curry can cause people to have bad breath. As you digest them, some of the elements flow through your bloodstream and to the lungs. The odor can be emitted for about 24 hours.

- Coffee and some teas can also be culprits of bad breath. Both have plenty of acid in them. Try not to drink so much of these beverages.

Drinking black tea has elements that keep bacteria away. Other teas that can help to prevent bad breath are green tea and peppermint tea. Tea can also get rid of bad breath that is caused by mucus. You only have to drink one cup per day for the odor to gradually dissipate.

Vitamins and Supplements

- If you're not consuming enough zinc, then you could possibly have bad breath. If you are deficient, you need to take no less than 60 mg a day. Be careful about taking too much of this as zinc can interfere with copper.

- The lack of Vitamin B can also be a cause of bad breath. You may want to take some niacinimide, a B complex tablet and Vitamin B6 one time a day.

- If you consume no more than 6,000 mg of Vitamin C, you will remove the mucus and toxins that have built up in your body. The mucus and toxins that are stored up in your body can be a cause of bad breath.

Digestive System

Your digestive system can also be a cause of bad breath. You will need to improve it by watching what you eat. What you eat is crucial because it will determine whether or not it will help to eliminate bad breath. Here are some things that you can do to keep your digestive system in tact:

- Have a high-fiber diet that includes whole grains, along with fresh fruits and vegetables. These foods usually digest better than those that are not high in fiber.
- If you don't have enough enzymes to digest properly, you need to take no more than four tablets of enzymes for each major meal.
- You may not have enough hydrochloric acid. To get more in your system, you can use apple cider vinegar. Take one tablespoon before you eat a major meal. You can also use betaine or pepsin tablets before you eat in order to help your digestive system to work.
- You can also get bad breath from lack of regular bowel movements (constipation). You need to drink at least eight glasses of water (eight ounces) every day.

Herbal Remedies

- Basil, rosemary, parsley and thyme can help to get rid of bad breath.
- Use alfalfa tablets to get rid of bad breath.
- A lemon wedge with salt can help you if you eat onions or garlic.
- Make tea with cloves. Use three whole ones or ground, combine it with hot water and let it sit for no more than 20 minutes.
- Fennel can be used to place on your gums and your tongue to get rid of bad breath.

Natural gum that has spearmint or peppermint oils is good to use for bad breath. Using these oils can eliminate the bacterium that causes bad breath. When you chew the gum, you produce saliva which gets rid of the bad breath.

- A South American remedy that is used is gargling with one teaspoon of honey and cinnamon powder. Combine the mixture with hot water. This should be done in the morning. It supposed to keep your breath fresh all day.

- Chewing sage can help you get rid of bad breath. Sage has oils that have an antibacterial element that helps to get rid of the foul odor.

- Peppermint can be used in tea to calm your stomach. You exhale through your lungs and your breath has a nice sweet smell to it.

- Tea tree oil comes from the Melaleuca plant. This oil has elements that can disinfect your mouth and get rid of the bacteria. Tea tree oil can be found in toothpaste.

For some people, using herbs can work better for their system because they are not abrasive to their system. Not only are they a natural product, but since these herbs are taken orally, they will affect your blood and eventually provide a relief for your bad breath.

Other things that you may take to eliminate bad breath may work, but they will also go through your entire body and all of your pores. Herbal remedies work not only for your bad breath, but they also work for your health.

Herbal remedies don't cover up the bad breath issue. They work to eliminate the problem. It works to pinpoint what is triggering your breath to smell bad. In order for herbal remedies to work properly, it has to correct and get rid of the problem.

Using herbal remedies can also help you to change the way you eat and what you eat. If you consume a lot of red meat or dairy products, you will have bad breath lingering until everything you've consumed has digested in your system.

Some people think it may only be a few minutes for the bad breath to stick around. However, that is far from the truth. Eating large amounts of food such as described above will not help you get rid of halitosis.

Chinese Herbs

Chinese medicines have been around for many years. People use them to cure certain ailments that they are afflicted with. A lot of those treatments use Chinese herbs. Tackling bad breath is no different.

Some of the herbs used to get rid of bad breath include bamboo leaves, honeysuckle and gypsum, just to name a few. These herbs have shown to be effective in combating bad breath. Since there are so many Chinese herbs, you will have to know which ones to use in order to get rid of bad breath.

If you're not sure of what to use, consult with your physician or ask someone who is familiar with Chinese herbs to provide you with a solution. You can also check online, but you probably will still need to consult with someone.

Breath Spray

Some people choose to use breath spray in order to get rid of bad breath. This remedy may work, then again it may not. If you have chronic halitosis, it could be some underlying cause that breath spray can't cure. Using breath spray is really a temporary fix. If your halitosis is caused from something internally, then breath spray will not help you.

If you are experiencing digestive problems along with bad breath, consult with a physician to see what the problem is. It may be something more serious than just bad breath.

Breath spray is ok to use if your bad breath is temporary. When you're looking for breath spray to use, look for that which doesn't contain any alcohol. Alcohol can work for you and against you. Even though it does get rid of bad breath bacteria, it is also known for dry mouth.

The latter can make your bad breath escalate even more.

Choosing the right breath spray is very important while you work to get rid of bad breath. Look for breath spray that is oil-based rather than alcohol based. The best kind of breath spray is that which contains peppermint or eucalyptus oil.

Even if you get a breath spray that has a minty smell, it may not take care of your bad breath. It will only work temporarily. In addition to using the right breath spray, make sure that you continue to practice good oral hygiene every day. That includes brushing and flossing after each meal. Doing this will help you to maintain your oral health and keep your bad breath from recurring.

Over The Counter Medications (OTC)

People that are looking for a quick fix for their bad breath will usually go to the drugstore to get an over the counter medication. That is usually the first thing that people think about. However, if you don't know much about the product, you have wasted time and money.

The drugstore carries plenty of medications that are used for bad breath. You don't need a prescription to get them. They are not all guaranteed to eliminate bad breath from your system.

Every case of bad breath is not the same and you may not know the root of why you have bad breath. There is more than one type of bad breath and each type may need different kind of treatment. If you don't know the specifics, then you may not be able to get rid of your bad breath like you want.

You may need to consult with your physician to see what you need to take in order to get rid of your bad breath. You may have to get something that is stronger and will be more effective than the over the counter medicine.

For the most part, the over the counter medications used to get rid of bad breath are not as powerful as the ones you are prescribed by your physician. People that purchase over the counter medications for bad breath use natural products.

They usually don't contain ingredients such as antibiotics. You usually get antibiotics through a prescription. Over the counter medication usually provides limited and temporary relief.

Before you purchase over the counter medications, consult with your physician to see if it would work for you. You physician will be able to determine what kind of remedy you will need to get rid of bad breath.

Using Flaxseed For Bad Breath

Flaxseed is important to use for people that have bad breath. However, you need to know the root cause of your bad breath. You must also look at how flaxseed is produced. Actually flaxseed would fare better for you than over the counter medications would.

Using flaxseed to get rid of bad breath can be used because of the Omega-3 properties it has. Omega-3 fatty acids can be used to get rid of bad breath.

Flaxseed has important oils that can provide nutrients to your body. It uses oils and supplements that your body can use to get rid of bath breath. Flaxseed can also be used if you're suffering from chronic halitosis. This is a good use for it because there are plenty of fatty acids that can fight the bacteria that cause bad breath.

Quick Remedies For Bad Breath

Are you one of those people that goes to a social event and within a moment, you're breath doesn't smell right? Or are you in a meeting and you're supposed to meet with one of the big wigs in the company? At these types of gatherings, it will be impossible to not talk. You will have to put on your thinking cap and find some quick remedies to get rid of your bad breath.

Here are some ways that you can save yourself from embarrassment:

- Drink water. Water can help to clean your mouth for a period of time. Your breath will be fresh. It will help you if you have to talk to someone on a moment's notice. Or if you feel you have dry mouth, then drink water to keep your mouth moist.

  Dry mouth and bad breath work hand in hand because of the bacteria that form inside. To give the water flavor, squeeze some juice from a lemon or a lime.

- Having a piece of candy or gum can also help you at the last minute. If you can find a piece, quickly put it in your mouth. Your breath will be fresh at least for that period of time. If you start talking, don't have the piece of candy swirling in your mouth.

- In addition to drinking water, you can also use water to rinse your mouth. If you do this on a regular basis.

- If you have a toothbrush handy, you can quickly brush your teeth and use clean tissue to wipe off the residue. This is a good strategy if you haven't made it to your destination and you're not near a rest room.

- You can quickly scrape your tongue with a scraper or a spoon. The thing about doing this is you will have to go somewhere in private. If you can find a bathroom, then you can attempt to do this. If you have any white spots on your tongue, remove them with the scraper or the spoon.

- If you don't have any mints or gum while you're out eating, you can eat the parsley that is used for decoration with your meal. Don't do this in front of anyone. Excuse yourself and go to the bathroom.

- Chew on the parsley for a few minutes. You may have to rinse out your mouth before you go back. You don't want people to see any green particles on your teeth.

- If you drink alcohol, you'll like this one. If you drink a small shot of whiskey, you can get away with getting rid of your bad breath for a while. It's been said that whiskey can get rid of germs that are on your teeth. This is not a promotion of drinking alcohol, but it's been said to work, so it's your choice whether or not you want to try this. The only caution is not to drink a lot of it, or you could become rather intoxicated.

When You Should Seek Medical Assistance

If you have bad breath that won't go away and you can't figure out why, or you have bad breath along with a health ailment, then you should consult a physician.

Let your physician know about your recurring bad breath and what you've been doing to combat it. The physician will ask you some questions. Some of the questions asked will be:

- What kind of odor or smell does your breath have? Fishy? Fruity? Funky? Alcohol?

- Do you eat spicy foods on a regular basis?

- Are you a smoker?

- Have you been practicing good oral hygiene?

- What kind of remedies have you tried for your bad breath?

- Are you having problems with your dental hygiene?

- Do you have any allergies, sinus problems, sore throat, etc.

- What other health issues are you experiencing?

Your physician will examine you. This will include checking your mouth and your nose. With a sore throat or mouth sores, they will need to get a culture.

Sometimes, they may order more tests to include:

- Chest x-ray

- Abdomen x-ray

- Endoscopy

- Testing (blood) for diabetes or renal (kidney) failure

If you have to see a dentist, they will check your mouth to see what's going on. In order to do that, your dentist may use an instrument to test for bad breath. One instrument that they use is called the halimeter.

A halimeter is a machine that records a reading of your breath using a tube. You blow into the tube as you would a breathalyzer machine. If you suspect that you have bad breath or chronic halitosis, your dentist may have you test your breath on a regular basis.

The dentist can also determine what is actually causing you to have bad breath. Some of them include hydrogen sulfide and dimethyl sulfide. When you know what chemicals are causing your unfortunate dilemma, you can make changes to what you do on a daily basis.

As your dentist sees what enzymes and chemicals are in your breath, they will be able to provide the proper treatment for your condition. The downside to these tests is that they can only be performed at the dentist's office.

In addition to the halimeter, your dentist may use other testing, such as gas chromatography and the BANA test, just to name a few.

How Smokers Can Get Rid Of Bad Breath

If you live with or are always around people who smoke, you probably don't care for the smell. You wouldn't want to be in close proximity with them either, because of their breath. A smoker's breath can smack you off of your feet, because it's so strong.

The bad breath from smoking cigarettes can linger for a long while, or it can be a constant thing, especially if they are chain smokers. Some people wish they could stay away, but they probably don't want to hurt the smoker's feelings.

However, there are things that smokers can do to relieve themselves and others of that strong cigarette odor:

- One of the best ways that a smoker can hide their bad breath from smoking is to chew gum. Get a flavor that is strong and will last a while. Or, you can chew sugar-free gum. Sugar-free gum is better for your teeth.

  Since your teeth and related areas can affect your breath, chewing gum is probably the easiest way to go. You can also get specialty gum that is designed just for smokers. However, this gum is a little costly.

- Get mints that have a long lasting flavor. They can last long enough until the smell goes away.

- One of the quickest ways to get rid of smoking breath is to brush your teeth. On the down side, it's impossible to always brush after you've smoked a cigarette. However, it can provide some help.

- Mouthwash is another way smokers can relieve themselves of bad breath. It can also provide some help, but it's difficult to use it after each time you've smoked.

- If you really want to get rid of nicotine breath, you should just kick the habit. Then, you can really work on keeping your breath fresh and getting rid of the bad breath. You will also regain your health. It may take a moment for the change to kick in, but at least you'll be free of smoke. It's also a good way to stop smoking.

How To Prevent Or Stop Bad Breath

As noted earlier in this report, chronic halitosis is caused by lack or regular oral hygiene. You have to brush and floss your teeth at least twice each day. If you already have bad breath, you can work to get rid of it by starting this regimen as soon as possible.

Flossing

Flossing is for cleaning your teeth in areas where your toothbrush cannot get to. Such areas include the pockets (the spaces between the teeth) and anywhere else where it is difficult for your toothbrush to reach.

You should floss first and then use your toothbrush. If you do the opposite, you may miss some spots between your teeth. Once they sit there, they can turn into plaque. If not removed in time, plaque will cause your teeth to rot and end up with periodontal or gum disease.

Flossing can remove food particles that were stuck in between your teeth while you were eating. Flossing can help you in your cardiovascular health as well as your dental health. Regular flossing can help prevent the onset of a stroke or heart attack. This is a very good reason why flossing should be part of anyone's daily dental hygiene routine.

In order to floss correctly, place the floss in the space between your teeth. Move the floss within the space using an up and down motion. The best way to remove the particles is to floss all of the sides of your teeth.

If you're not sure what to use, your dentist or dental assistant will be able to help you find the right flossing tool for your teeth. There are various kinds of floss available. You can get waxes or unwaxed floss.

There are different strengths such as super thin and super strong. You can also get floss that is flavored with peppermint or regular mint if that's what you want. You can also use dental floss holders if you need something sturdy to hold the floss in.

When you go to the dentist for a checkup, you can get complimentary floss from them. Waxed floss is better for you because it is easier to use. Along with that, your breath can smell minty fresh with the flavored wax.

Brushing

When you brush your teeth, it has to be done the right way. You can't just go over them once and think that's it. A lot of people don't take the time to brush their teeth properly. Doing this can leave particles in their teeth that may be difficult to get out, even with flossing.

Nowadays, people are so busy that they don't have time to hardly brush their teeth. Doing it too quickly can also lead to bacteria and plaque setting in. This can lead to other dental problems down the road.

The proper way to brush your teeth is to have your toothbrush at an angle of 45 degrees. You start brushing from the bottom going upward. You would start with your lower gums going upward to the top of your lower teeth.

Then you would brush downward from the top of the lower teeth. You should also brush your teeth on the outside using the same method. Brushing in this manner will help to move the plaque from your gums.

When plaque hits your gums, it can cause gum disease. Also brush where you chew in a horizontal direction. Finally, brush the chewing surfaces of your teeth with a horizontal movement.

In order to see results, you must make sure that you floss and brush on a regular basis every day. If you don't, your chances of getting rid of bad breath are slim.

Using Tongue Brushing To Get Rid Of Bad Breath

You can also brush your tongue to get rid of bad breath. In order to see results, you must do it correctly. You can use a toothbrush to do this. There are also other instruments you can buy that are used for tongue brushing. It should not be something abrasive where you would lose your taste buds.

The way to properly brush your tongue is to take your toothbrush or instrument and go the back of your tongue. Go back as far as you can. You may cough up and gag a little. However, this is the area that you want to focus on. A lot of the bacteria and germs are on the back of your tongue. When you brush, make sure to include the sides of your tongue.

After you have finished brushing your tongue, rinse your mouth several times. You must do a thorough job on this. You must get rid of the entire residue that remains in your mouth. That includes any food particles that you didn't get the first go round.

If you are going to implement tongue brushing, you should do it every time you brush your teeth. If you can't do that, at least do it once a day. You don't have to scrub your tongue; a few brushes with the toothbrush or tongue scraper will work.

Don't forget about your regular oral hygiene. Be sure to floss every day and stay away from foods that have lots of acid in them. Acidic foods tend to eliminate the enamel on your teeth.

When you rinse your mouth, use a solution that does not have alcohol. Tongue brushing would be for naught if you didn't implement regular oral hygiene. You will start to see results once you implement these changes on a regular basis.

How To Help Others That Have Bad Breath

Children That Have Bad Breath

Having bad breath is not just limited to adults. Children have to deal with chronic halitosis as well. However, they don't have as many causes to deal with like adults would. Still, parents need to find out the root cause because once other children find out, they will start to tease and distance themselves from the child who is afflicted with bad breath.

Usually, the cause of bad breath in children is not having the proper dental hygiene. If they're not monitored while brushing their teeth, then either they don't brush them correctly, or they won't brush them at all.

They can leave food particles in their mouth and then if it stays there, it turns into bacteria. It mixes in with the saliva in your mouth and that's what causes the child to have bad breath.

If your children don't brush their teeth regularly, then they will have bad breath for the rest of the day. Just like adults, children should brush their teeth once in the morning and once before they go to bed at night.

They can also have cavities. If the cavity is superficial, it can cause the child to have bad breath. Or they can have allergies. As with adults, children have allergies as well. They can have sinusitis or a throat infection.

A child can experience sinus problems when mucus clogs into the pharynx. They may have a dry cough where it keeps them up at night. Along with that, their eyes will itch and they can have a runny nose.

Parents are responsible for making sure that their children learn proper oral hygiene. They must advise their child on the proper way to brush their teeth. Stress to the child (or children) how important is it for them to keep their teeth clean every day.

If the child is young, it is not advisable for them to use mouthwash for their teeth. It may not be effective in getting their teeth clean. In addition to that, regular mouthwash has alcohol which might prove to be too strong for them to use anyway.

You can check with your child (or children) to make sure that they are brushing their teeth the proper way. Show them how they are supposed to brush their teeth. Take them to the dentist at least every six months to once a year. When they start going at a young age, they will learn to take care of their teeth better.

The Date With Bad Breath

How would you feel if you went on a date, they started talking to you and out came a whiff of a foul odor? You would be taken aback, wouldn't you? Depending on your personality, you may or may not say anything. However, that may be the last date that you have with them.

If you are going on a date, it's important for your breath to be free of any foul odors. If you suffer from chronic halitosis, you will need to correct the problem before you meet that person. You probably wouldn't want to talk to anyone either if you had this problem.

If you're at the kissing stage, it is a must that your breath is fresh. Not having a fresh breath can turn off your date. They probably will not want to go out with you again. It can also work the other way around. You may not want to go out with them again.

You have to work at keeping your breath fresh, especially if you have chronic halitosis. If you don't implement regular oral hygiene, now is the time to do so. If you don't, you can forget about going on dates with anyone else for a while.

If you are a smoker that dates, you need to keep gum or mints on you at all times. A smoker's breath is one of the worst ones to smell. Not only is it strong, if it is not corrected, can last a while in your mouth. If you are a chain smoker, this horrid smoke breath will definitely last.

On the other hand, you may be on a date and not know that you have bad breath. It's not like you get up in the morning and decide to test it. There may be someone in your circle who is brave enough to tell you about it.

Or if your date has bad breath, you may be livid to let them know what's going on. However, you may have to be brave and tell them about it. They may not know that their breath has an odor.

If you're the one with the bad breath, your date may feel the same way, so they decide not to go out with you again. They'll leave you wondering why and you may never know. Whichever way it goes, telling a date about their bad breath is not an easy task.

How To Tell A Friend Or Family Member

Everyone has some type of personal problem that they are dealing with. Some are more serious than others. When it comes to bad breath, that is considered a serious problem. Having bad breath will keep people away from you.

It will be difficult to maintain a social life, because people will be offended by your foul breath odor. There are some people who just don't feel that they can come out and tell you what's wrong. They feel that you may take it the wrong way.

The ways that people deal with something such as bad breath are different. Even if you say it the right way, there are some people who are really sensitive and will really take it to heart and feel offended.

There are ways to deliver what you have to say in a professional and tactful manner. You have to do it in a way where your friend or relative will understand that you care and you're not trying to hurt them.

You should not sound abrasive or brash when you're talking to them. There are some things that you should not say to them, no matter what:

- Asking them when was the last time they brushed their teeth.

- Telling them outright that their breath stinks.

- Emphasizing to them that their breath stinks.

- Constantly repeating to them that their breath stinks.

- Making gestures that in front of them that they would be easily offended by.

Be considerate of their feelings. They may be going through some other things and you telling them outright that their breath stinks don't make it any better. People already feel bad about the insecurities that they do have. Adding something like this could ignite more flames.

You can talk to them like you normally do in a conversation. Then you can ask them if they've had any issues with their oral health. You can set the tone so where they will feel comfortable talking to you about it.

You may get one of three responses: Yes, No, or they don't want to talk about it. If it's yes, see if they want to explore the subject some more. If the answer is no, then maybe you can talk to them about halitosis.

If they know and are not willing to discuss it with you, then wait for a time when they feel comfortable discussing it.

If you do get to speak with them about it, let them know that this is related to their health. It's not just a regular health issue, it's also a dental hygiene issue. Let them know that they can seek help from a physican, a dentist or both.

Let them know about regular brushing and flossing of their teeth. They need to know that it's very important that they brush and floss on a regular basis. They also need to know the purpose of doing this so they can get rid of their bad breath.

Also let them know they can be left out socially f they don't take care of their oral hygiene. If you're able to get this message across to them without them being offended, then you're off to a good start. Don't hesitate to offer additional assistance if needed.

Resources

American Dental Association, http://www.ada.org/public/topics/bad_breath.asp

National Institutes Of Health (Medline Plus),
http://www.nlm.nih.gov/medlineplus/ency/article/003058.htm

About.com

http://healing.about.com/od/ritalouise/a/badbreath_RL.htm

http://babyparenting.about.com/od/healthandsafety/a/badbreath.htm

http://pediatrics.about.com/od/weeklyquestion/a/05_bad_breath.htm

http://adam.about.com/encyclopedia/Breath-odor.htm

http://dentistry.about.com/od/dentalhealth/Basic_Dental_Care_Brushing_Flossing_Dental_Check_ups.htm (has a listing of articles regarding dental care)

Mayo Clinic, http://mayoclinic.com/health/bad-breath/DS00025

Centers For Disease Control (CDC),
http://www2a.cdc.gov/podcasts/player.asp?f=9405

This is a podcast about periodontal disease and diabetes.

Printed in Great Britain by
Amazon.co.uk, Ltd.,
Marston Gate.